Order from
 Research Corp.
 405 Sellington Ave
 N.Y., N.Y. 10017
 Free

D1346555

A Practical Guide
to Combating Malnutrition
in the Preschool Child

A Practical Guide to Combating Malnutrition in the Preschool Child

Nutritional Rehabilitation through Maternal Education

Report of a Working Conference
on Nutritional Rehabilitation or Mothercraft Centers
National Institute of Nutrition,
Bogota, Colombia, March 1969

Sponsored by Research Corporation

Appleton-Century-Crofts
Educational Division
Meredith Corporation
New York

Library of Congress Catalog Card Number: 77-127-202

SBN 390 73346 6

Cover Illustration: Picasso—Mother and Child—1904.

Lithograph—courtesy Harlem Book Company
Division of Computer Applications Incorporated,
New York

Printed in the United States of America

Produced by William Bennett and Maura Fitzgerald

National Institute of Nutrition of Colombia
**Working Conference
on Nutritional Rehabilitation or Mothercraft Centers**
Sponsored by Research Corporation, March 17-21, 1969

Conference President and Chairman:
Dr. Roberto Rueda-Williamson
Honorary Chairman:
Dr. W. Henry Sebrell, Jr.
General Secretariat:
Dr. Jaime Ariza-Macias
Dr. Kendall W. King
Dr. Francisco Piedrahita
Editorial Advisor:
Richard S. Baldwin,
Assistant to the President, Research Corporation

Participants

Brazil

Dr. Ivan D. Beghin
Pan American Health Organization
Caixa Postal 2643
Recife, Brazil

Colombia

Dr. Jaime Ariza-Macias
National Institute of Nutrition
Apartado Aereo 15.609
Bogota, Colombia

Dr. Harrison E. McKay
Department of Nutrition
Faculty of Medicine
University of Valle
Cali, Colombia

Dr. Jaime Paez
National Institute of Nutrition
Apartado Aereo 15.609
Bogota, Colombia

Dr. Francisco Piedrahita
Ministry of Health
Bogota, Colombia

Dr. Roberto Rueda-Williamson
National Institute of Nutrition
Apartado Aereo 15.609
Bogota, Colombia

Dr. Leonardo Sinisterra
Department of Nutrition
Faculty of Medicine
University of Valle
Cali, Colombia

Costa Rica

Dr. Carlos Diaz Amador
Ministry of Health
Republic of Costa Rica
San Jose, Costa Rica

Guatemala

Dr. Romeo de Leon
Nutrition Department,
Office of Director of Public Health
Guatemala City, Guatemala

Dr. Otto Retana
Institute of Nutrition
for Central America and Panama
Carretera Roosevelt Zona 11
Guatemala City, Guatemala

Haiti

Dr. Warren L. Berggren
Hopital Albert Schweitzer
P. O. Box #2213-B
Port-au-Prince, Haiti

Participants

Miss Gladys Dominique
Bureau of Nutrition
P. O. Box 707
Port-au-Prince, Haiti

Dr. William Fougere
Bureau of Nutrition
P. O. Box 707
Port-au-Prince, Haiti

Mrs. Linda D. Gonzales
Bureau of Nutrition
P. O. Box 707
Port-au-Prince, Haiti

Peru

Dr. Mario Eisler
Pan American Health Organization
Casilla Postal 2117, Zona IV
Lima, Peru

Philippines

Dr. R. W. Engel
U. S. Agency
for International Development
1680 Roxas Boulevard
Manila, Philippines

Dr. Lourdes M. Sumabat
National Nutrition Program
Department of Health
Republic of the Philippines

Mrs. Dwayne Suter
Methodist Mission
San Mateo, Isabela Province
Republic of the Philippines

Switzerland

Dr. Jose Maria Bengoa
Nutrition Section
World Health Organization
1211 Geneva 27, Switzerland

United States

Dr. Kendall W. King
Research Corporation
405 Lexington Avenue
New York, New York, 10017

Dr. W. Henry Sebrell, Jr.
Institute of Nutrition Sciences
Columbia University
511 West 166 Street
New York, New York 10032

Dr. Sam C. Smith
Research Corporation
405 Lexington Avenue
New York, New York 10017

Venezuela

Dr. Hernan Mendez-Castellano
Rehabilitation Unit
National Institute of Nutrition
Apartado 2049
Caracas, Venezuela

Contents

Contents

Foreword

Malnutrition is the single most extensive and serious public health problem affecting the preschool child in the world today. Yet in every nation where it exists there are concerned people —professional and lay—who will work toward its eradication if they are convinced that their efforts will bring results.

This book is intended as a practical guide for organizations and individuals who are aware of the problem, who recognize that, while the final solution may be years away, it is essential to mount an attack *now* to cut down the appalling death, suffering, and loss of human potential caused by malnutrition.

The authors of this volume are 23 scientists, physicians, nutritionists, and activists who have planned, established, operated, and evaluated Nutritional Rehabilitation or Mothercraft Centers in most of the nations where such Centers now exist. They drafted the text at a working conference held at the National Institute of Nutrition, Bogota, Colombia in March 1969 under the sponsorship of Research Corporation.

I had the privilege of welcoming the conferees in Bogota on behalf of the sponsoring foundation, of observing the formal presentations, and of talking with the authors at a number of informal sessions. Both in their papers and their personal comments I was struck by the wide diversity in methods of Center operation, but even more by the greater commonness of purpose.

One Center in Venezuela is in an urban area, handsomely housed in a modern building with a well-equipped kitchen. It is closely linked physically and functionally with a complete range of health and medical services from an out-patient clinic to pediatric beds in a hospital.

Another Center in Haiti, in a remote rural region, operates in a village hut where the cooking is done in family-type utensils over a charcoal fire on an earthen table-stove. Its nearest medical facility is hours away, and only a modicum of professional guidance and help is available through periodic visits of a physician or nutritionist.

As is made abundantly clear in the pages of this book, both of these Centers—and many other possible variations—are founded on a single concept: educating mothers in child care by involving them in the nutritional rehabilitation of their own children, using foods, facilities, and methods that are within their financial means and their ability to comprehend.

Research Corporation is deeply indebted to the conferees, all of whom interrupted their own important work to prepare for and attend the Bogota meetings and to write this volume; to the National Institute of Nutrition of Colombia which made available its excellent facilities, staff, and services; and most especially to its Director at that time, Dr. Roberto Rueda-Williamson, President and Chairman of the conference and its gracious host, and Dr. W. Henry Sebrell, Jr., Honorary Chairman of the conference.

In this book is the essence of the accumulated knowledge and experience of most of the people who are the leaders today in nutritional rehabilitation through maternal education. The guidelines are purposely broad so that the concept can be adapted to the widest variations in local conditions; references are included for more detailed and more specific data.

Beyond this, all of the participants and authors have offered to furnish information or advice, or to contribute in any other way they can, to anyone who wishes to take part in similar efforts. It is their hope, and ours, that this book will serve as a stimulus and a working blueprint to many new actions to attack the scourge of infant malnutrition at its source—maternal ignorance.

James S. Coles
President, Research Corporation

January 5, 1970

1

A New Attack on Child Malnutrition

A child's entire life is determined in large measure by the food his mother gives him during his first five years. A serious dietary deficiency will damage his health, inhibit his growth, and possibly impair his mental development. He may not live to see his sixth birthday and, if he should survive, he may very well carry the scars throughout his life.

Not only is this a personal tragedy for the damaged child and his family, but—multiplied by millions—its cultural and economic impact on national development is appalling. No nation can afford a generation of men and women incapable of functioning in accordance with its genetic potential.

1

In some of the developing countries one child out of every four below the age of five is so severely malnourished as to need urgent attention. This age group accounts for one-fourth to one-half of all deaths—twenty to thirty times the toll taken in the industrialized nations.

Malnutrition alone is often not the immediate cause of death, but its debilitating effects render far more deadly the common infectious diseases of childhood, such as gastroenteritis, measles, and respiratory ailments.

The Long-Term Solution

The most desirable and lasting solution to the problem depends upon long-term measures aimed at social and economic development. Sustained efforts are needed to improve sanitation, increase the availability of proper foods, expand the purchasing power of families, and raise their educational levels.

Preventive programs are also required to maintain the status of well-nourished children and to reduce the incidence and the effects of infectious diseases. Special emphasis is needed on development of new low-cost protein-rich foods, the formulation of indigenous preparations for infant feeding, the education of mothers in the least-cost adequate feeding of their children, and the extension of immunization programs.

Because the best solution calls for the motivation of so many people—with attendant profound changes in their way of life—and for very large capital investments, these efforts must necessarily be carried on for long periods of time before their impact becomes noticeable. Meanwhile, and for many years to come, there will inevitably be vast numbers of preschool-age children whose poor nutritional status will call for immediate and specific attention.

Shortcomings of Past Approaches

Welfare-type supplementary feeding programs, though urgently needed at times for humanitarian and practical reasons, do not correct the causes of malnutrition. Effective nutrition education must be conducted if a lasting improvement in the health of the world's children is ever to be realized.

The idea that the malnourished child requires hospitalization is still very widespread. And yet, while there are remarkable exceptions, hospital facilities in developing countries are woefully inadequate to handle the number of malnourished children needing attention. In one of these countries it is reliably estimated that there are 23,000 cases of kwashiorkor in infants on any given day, but there are only about 130 pediatric beds in the whole nation. Further, hospitalization of malnourished children is a tremendous economic burden which absorbs human and financial resources that could generally be channeled to more efficient ways of combating malnutrition.

While it is obvious that extremely severe cases—particularly those with complications—should have hospital care, it is now known that a large proportion of the advanced cases of malnutrition requires simply a proper diet for successful recuperation. Even when hospitalization can be provided and the child is successfully treated, many cases eventually relapse because treatment alone fails to correct the underlying causes of his illness, which lie in his own home.

An important reason for such relapses is the ignorance on the part of mothers of the nutritional and sanitary needs of their children. Instruction of mothers having a limited background of formal education is not a simple task. To be successful, teaching techniques must be used which are compatible with their current understanding, their educational background, and their food and financial resources.

The Center Concept

The Centers which are described here in various modifications were developed primarily to educate mothers of malnourished children and secondarily to rehabilitate the children at a substantially lower cost than in hospitals. Dr. Jose Maria Bengoa, on the basis of his earlier experience as a physician in rural Venezuela, proposed the establishment of such Centers in 1955. Since then a number of countries, including Algeria, Brazil, Colombia, Costa Rica, Ecuador, Guatemala, Haiti, Nigeria, Peru, The Philippines, Uganda, and Venezuela, have set up Nutritional Rehabilitation or Mothercraft Centers. Most are found in Latin America, and in Colombia, Guatemala, and Haiti they constitute nationwide efforts.

A number of different names are used to describe the Centers: Nutritional Rehabilitation Centers, Nutritional Recuperation Centers, Nutrition Education and Recuperation Centers, Nutrition Education and Recuperation Services, and Mothercraft Centers. While there are certain differences in emphasis and operation, they are all fundamentally similar in that they share the same philosophy and objectives. The differences in names reflect primarily local preferences.

Education and Recuperation. The main purpose of a Center is to educate the mother through her active participation in the nutritional recuperation of her child in order to reduce morbidity and mortality, and to permit realization of the genetic potentiality for growth and development of her children.

The first objective is to provide nutrition education for the mother and thereby to improve her capacity to care for her children; concurrently the nutritional recuperation of her malnourished child is brought about by the use of an adequate diet of inexpensive locally available foods. If the mother does not apply at home what she learned at the Center, her child can be expected to relapse when he leaves the Center, and there will be no permanent improvement in his nutritional status nor in that of her other children.

Centers combine child day-care and maternal education with the serving of a well-balanced diet of local foods carefully planned to meet the nutritional requirements of preschool children at minimum cost. A Center that provides full daily dietary needs for six days a week, including holidays, can over a three- to four-month period recuperate most children—even those suffering from relatively severe malnutrition.

Mothers are assigned responsibilities at the Centers, with each participating at regular intervals over the full period her child is there. The assignments include selecting, preparing, and serving food to the children, and taking part in other educational activities. Mothers serve full days on a rotation basis so that there is always one mother to every five or six children at the Center. From 25 to 30 children and five or six mothers constitute a cohesive and manageable group.

The mothers' education involves not only demonstrations and participation in practical nutrition, but the elements of personal hygiene and good sanitary practices as well. They are taught— along with their children—to use the Center's toilet facilities, to observe basic rules of personal cleanliness, and to avoid contamination of food. If their education is successful, they make these practices a part of their life at home.

The Center may or may not be attached to a health facility, and it may in some cases admit children overnight. These decisions depend on local circumstances, as do the degree and extent to which other community activities are associated with the Center.

As a rule, the Center is housed and operated in a way that is as close as possible to the conditions prevailing in the community. It uses the same type of housing, cooking utensils, fuel, and furniture as those found in local homes.

Low-Cost Operation. A fundamental principle of the Center is operation at a very low cost in comparison with the cost of treatment in a hospital. Figures collected from eight Centers in five Latin American countries show that the cost of operating a Center of the day-care type is 50 to 75 cents (U.S.) per child per day, of which food and fuel account for 13 to 44 cents. Food and fuel costs vary considerably since they should approximate the amount the mothers will have to spend on these items when they return home with their children.

These costs generally are only one-seventh to one-tenth of the average expense for hospital care which does not provide education for the mothers. Some Centers report still lower food costs, and in several countries the difference between the cost of operating a Center and the cost of hospitalization is even larger. In a well-run Center a severely malnourished child can be recuperated—and his mother educated well enough to prevent his relapse and to forestall the onset of malnutrition in her other children—for a total cost of no more than $50 (U.S.).

While malnourished children may also be recuperated through even less expensive means, such as supplemental feeding or long-range nutrition education programs not providing Center-type care for the children, the time needed to achieve recuperation is usually much longer, and during this time the children may be exposed to additional risks from infectious diseases. Supplemental feeding programs, as well as solely educational activities, also require very close supervision at the child's home if they are to be effective.

Other Health Benefits. While a Center's prime role is that of nutritional rehabilitation through maternal education, it can bring additional health benefits to the community. Public health personnel and other community workers can be trained in effective techniques of public health nutrition and community development. Information on proper infant feeding practices can be disseminated to the community as a whole, not just to the mothers in attendance. A Center can receive partially re-cuperated children from hospitals, thereby freeing beds in pediatric wards and reducing recuperation costs.

The organization and operation of Centers should not be considered as an isolated program, and certainly not as a single complete solution to the problem of child malnutrition. A Center should be thought of as one link in the chain of activities that are needed for the eventual eradication of malnutrition. It is, however, a vital link in that chain, one that can bring immediate benefits while other longer-range improvements are being worked out.

Organizing for Action

Centers cannot operate in a vacuum. They should be integral parts of the maternal and child-care branch of medical and health services, such as hospitals, health units, and stations, that are available to the population. The type of organization that is evolved for the Centers will, therefore, depend to a large degree on the availability of such services. However, Centers have been operated very effectively where these medical and para-medical programs did not exist and, in some instances, the Centers have led to the establishment of more sophisticated health services.

For the operation of a network of Centers a central staff is needed to insure uniform planning and control of field operations, and to provide professional and technical support for the whole program. This staff may be a part of the maternal and child welfare services, or a separate entity.

The structure of the headquarters staff will, of course, vary with local conditions and availability of other health services. Appendix I gives examples of three different types of organizations that have proved to be practical in the countries where Centers have been established. Whatever its form, however, the central organization is responsible for:

Establishing norms, such as height-weight standards or nutrient intake goals, for nutritional rehabilitation and prevention of malnutrition.

Selecting and training personnel to operate and supervise the Centers.

Providing equipment, materials, and supplies, and distributing them to the Centers.

Evaluating Center operations to determine their effectiveness and to apply corrective measures as necessary.

Coordinating with other agencies in identifying the factors responsible for infant malnutrition and seeking solutions for long-range improvement.

The minimum requirement for the headquarters staff is a director or principal administrative officer. The director should be a physician with a strong interest and sound knowledge in nutrition, or a person with an advanced degree in nutrition. In either case it is important that this officer have leadership and administrative capabilities.

A suggested additional central staff professional is an assistant director whose functions would include selection, training, and development of personnel, general supervision of the Centers, and interpretation and evaluation of data collected in field operations. This person should be a qualified nutritionist-dietitian, preferably with some experience in public health nutrition.

Where feasible, a third professional staff member is desirable, also a nutritionist-dietitian, who has a genuine appreciation of food economics, so as to be able to develop least-cost adequate diets. This person would have specific responsibility for working out recipes and menu cycles, calculating their nutrient content, and testing their acceptability.

Field Support Staff

The minimum requirement for the field support staff is a physician and a nutritionist-dietitian. If possible, there should also be a public health nurse.

The physician should be trained in public health, pediatrics, or clinical nutrition. If the Centers are integrated with existing health services, the physician at the health station could be responsible for medical control of the children as a part of the out-patient clinic services. If the Center is not a part of the health services, a physician with the necessary qualifications will be needed on a part-time basis, with a minimum of one day a week devoted to medical support of field operations.

Functions of the physician will include selecting children to be admitted to the Center after clinical examination, providing medical care or arranging hospital treatment for children referred by the Centers, and deciding the proper time for discharge of children from the Centers. In addition, the physician should help with appropriate teaching activities of the Centers and in evaluating the effectiveness of their operation.

The nutritionist-dietitian should have the qualifications rec-

ommended at the Pan American Health Organization Confer-
ence on Nutritionist-Dietitian Training held in Caracas in 1967.*
More than one may be needed, depending on the number of
Centers operating and their distance from the central office.
There should be enough nutritionist-dietitians to allow at least
one visit per week to each Center.

Functions of the nutritionist-dietitian include overall supervision of a group of Centers, helping to select and train personnel for the Centers, determining least-cost local foods,
making up menus, substitutions, and market lists, and evaluating the children's acceptance of recipes. Other functions are
developing educational material and assisting in teaching the
mothers, helping to evaluate the Centers' effectiveness, and coordinating the Centers' work with that of other related agencies.
The nutritionist-dietitian cooperates with Center managers in
the preparation of reports on Center operations.

The public health nurse, if available, should have as minimum qualification a bachelor's degree in nursing with special
training in public health, along with capability for establishing
good rapport with the mothers. Like the physician, the nurse
may or may not be on the staff of a health center; in any event
she should be available one day a week.

The functions of the nurse are similar to those of the nutritionist-dietitian in working with Center personnel, in teaching,
evaluation, and coordination with other agencies. In addition,
she should be able to perform immunizations and to follow up
on the progress of children discharged by the Centers.

Center Staff

The minimum requirement for each Center is a manager, a
cook, and a nurse's aid or helper, if sufficient mothers are not

---

* The proceedings of this conference may be obtained from the Pan American
Health Organization, Washington, D.C.

available on a regular basis. In some instances a mother may serve as the cook.

The Manager. The manager is the person in charge, and as such may be given any title that is suitable in the circumstances. She may be an auxiliary nurse, teacher, or equivalent, if available. Preferably she should have had twelve years of schooling, but the minimum educational level acceptable should be six to eight years of school. The theoretical and practical training she needs will vary with her background and previous training, but generally two weeks of intensive instruction and two weeks of practical work in the field will be sufficient. When placed in charge of a Center, she has a full-time job with responsibilities in three major areas: administrative, educational, and paramedical.

The manager's administrative duties include the setting of schedules for mothers' attendance at the Center, purchasing food with the help of the mothers, and supervising the feeding of the children. Among the daily records she must keep are clinical reports, menu cycles, expenditures, and attendance of children and mothers. She is also responsible for such household chores as checking on the condition of equipment and overseeing the routine cleaning. In the event of an epidemic in the community causing the Center to suspend temporarily, she will arrange to have the food distributed to the families to assure continuity of the program.

Educational activities of the manager follow a schedule set by the headquarters office. In general she will teach the mothers elementary principles of foods and nutrition as related to the most economic use of the family food budget. She will counsel mothers on the duration of breast feeding and the use of infant food supplements and weaning foods, and instruct them on sanitation, hygiene, and other elements of child care.

Paramedical and other activities for which the manager is

responsible include the reception and inspection of the children, looking after their personal hygiene, applying first-aid measures as necessary, and referring to the physician any child with suspected illness. Most important, she will keep a careful periodic register of weight and height of all children attending the Center, generally taking the weights weekly or biweekly and the heights monthly. She will keep the individual performance charts and health records, as well as the attendance records of mothers and children. Among her other responsibilities are the development and supervision of recreational and educational activities for the children in the Center and making visits to their homes.

The Cook.   The cook should be someone from the local community with ordinary cooking skills who is capable of following recipe instructions and preparing meals as specified by the menus furnished. She may be one of the mothers, but she must be available on a full-time basis for duty in the Center.

The cook's functions include preparation of meals, proper storage and conservation of food, and assistance to the supervisor in teaching food handling and cooking techniques. Among her housekeeping duties are caring for cooking utensils and keeping the kitchen clean.

The Helper.   The nurse's aid or helper, if mothers are not available for this function on a regular basis, should be someone from the community who can work comfortably with the children and mothers. She will help serve the meals, feed the children and wash the dishes, as well as bathe the children and care for their personal hygiene, including assistance in use of toilet facilities. She will also help the supervisor with any recreational and educational activities of the children.

Equipping the Center

Equipment, materials, and supplies needed at the Center vary with the extent of self-help generated in the community and with the local customs. Following are some general guidelines to the kinds of items that will have to be provided to equip the Center for operation.

Equipment.   It is essential that all the necessary equipment be ready in the Center from the first day of its operation. The basic rules in its selection are simplicity and efficiency, especially for the kitchen equipment.

Since the ultimate purpose of the Center is to teach practices that can be duplicated in the children's homes, the kitchen equipment must be approximately the same as that commonly used in the community. The use of familiar utensils and facilities will increase the mothers' confidence and stimulate them to continue in their own homes the practices they learn at the Center.

The Center must also have its own equipment for making precise weight and height measurements of the children, for it is through these parameters that a large part of the success of the Center will be judged.

Appendix II contains detailed equipment lists for Centers of two different types tailored to the standards of living of the mothers being taught; these may serve as rough guides, but it is extremely important that in any community the equipment provided be familiar to the mothers.

Materials and Supplies.   Materials and supplies for feeding the children are the recommended local foods, including condiments, fuel for cooking, and copies of menu cycles and recipes. (Appendix III gives examples of recipes that are based on traditional, well-accepted dishes in several different countries.) First-aid supplies are also needed, as are appropriate nursery supplies and inexpensive pads or matting for rest and naps.

Among educational materials to aid in teaching the mothers are simplified illustrations of the three or four classes from which foods can be selected for least-cost menus. Elaborate or complex educational materials should be avoided, as they may confuse or discourage the mothers. Growth charts of the children, prominently displayed, will show graphically the nutritional rehabilitation of the children and will lend incentive.

A few standardized forms will simplify the keeping of the Center's records; examples are the individual performance charts and health records shown in Appendixes IV and VI. These and the attendance records are important for the supervision of Center operation. Other useful forms are those used for noting individual eating habits and for collecting food habit data, including weaning practices.

Items that will help in the motivation of the community, as well as in maintaining the mothers' interest in good nutrition after they leave the Center, are useful but not critical. Photos of the children taken on their admittance and again on their discharge will give the mothers permanent proof of the Center's work. Certificates awarded to mothers who have completed their training at the Centers are almost certain to be displayed proudly in the homes; they are good reminders to the mothers to continue to apply their newly acquired knowledge on child care.

Coordinating with Other Programs

As indicated earlier, Centers are integrated with such other health and medical resources as are available. Similarly, in order to have an impact on long-range solutions to the problem of malnutrition, they should be coordinated with other community development agencies and programs operating in their areas.

Among such agencies and programs are those dealing with social welfare, handicrafts, agricultural extension efforts, community cooperatives, and credit institutions. An excellent reference for further information is a United Nations publication, which describes how agriculture, education, community development, and health services can be coordinated with

Center-type operations to produce a total community nutrition-education program.*

Working with the appropriate agencies and programs, Centers will emerge as a vital link, but not necessarily the best or ultimate answer to overcoming malnutrition in early childhood. Contributions to long-range results, however, can be made by also utilizing Centers for such applied research as the testing of new protein-rich food products or weaning foods. A network of Centers can also serve in experimental programs, with adequate controls, such as the impact of de-worming versus no treatment on children's response to nutritional rehabilitation.

Support of Centers

Still other agencies and organizations may also be interested in supporting or helping with actual Center operation. As shown in the examples in Appendix I, depending on the availability of health and medical services, Centers may be operated by the national organization, as in Colombia; by other interested groups, as in the Philippines; or by a combination of both, as in Haiti. Among the kinds of agencies and organizations whose support or help may be enlisted are universities, social welfare departments, education departments, church and civic groups, service clubs, voluntary organizations and others.

Because malnutrition is a disease, Centers should be organized in collaboration with the health and medical services where they are available, but this does not foreclose the opportunity for other groups to participate. Support by nonmedical groups can take many forms and can be useful even where there are excellent medical and health facilities. Where these facilities are less well developed, or virtually nonexistent, the support of other organizations may be critical in establishing and operating Centers. Success ultimately depends upon the ingenuity, persuasiveness, and cooperation of all concerned.

---

* This publication is WHO Tech. Rep. Ser. #340—1966 and may be obtained from World Health Organization, Geneva, Switzerland.

3

Locating the Center

The selection of the community in which a Center is to be established can in some cases be made on the basis of the obvious needs of a particular locality. In other instances a choice may have to be made among a number of communities which need help. Following are some of the major factors to be considered in making the selection.

Selecting the Community

Frequency of Malnutrition. Only communities with relatively high proportions of preschool children suffering from second-

and third-degree malnutrition should be selected for Center operations. Appendix VII describes the Gomez classification, one widely used to describe these advanced stages of malnutrition. The professional judgment of a physician trained in public health nutrition is helpful in making the final determination.

Availability of Medical Services. Whenever possible, the Center should be established in a community where health or medical services are available. These facilities can provide medical records of the children and other valuable information on the community's health needs, as well as the possibility of medical supervision by the physician who can refer complicated cases for hospital care or emergency medication. Such services can also be effective in helping to follow the progress of children discharged from the Center. In addition, there is a psychological advantage in being associated with an established institution that is known to the community as a source of medical and health care, and there are mutual benefits in centralization and sharing of resources and services between the Center and the medical or health group.

Where there is a choice, it is clear that a community with such existing services should be chosen over one without them. Yet there are many communities that do not have these services and which have needs which can be met through the establishment of Centers. In these situations, preliminary information about the health needs of the community can be gained by weighing all preschool children and checking their weights against the standards shown in Appendix VIII. There are also indirect indicators, such as death and sickness rates of children under five.

Daily, professional, medical supervision and immediate availability of hospital care for complicated cases are not necessities for the successful operation of a Center, and their absence in the face of a demonstrated need should not stand in the way of establishing a Center. It is important, however, that medical supervision and periodic visits by a physician be available.

Availability of Financial Resources. Before a Center can be established there must be adequate financial resources at hand to cover a reasonable period of time of its operation. Funds may be sought from interested public or private sources, or both. Whenever possible, the community itself should provide major contributions.

Accessibility and Concentration of Population. The total number of people in a community and the geographic area over which they are spread are important considerations in selecting a site for Center operations. Larger populations and greater concentrations should be given higher priority than smaller groups or those scattered over wide areas.

Economic Potential of the Community. Priority should be given to communities with the potential for attaining an economic or agricultural level compatible with least-cost minimum diets. In a community with little or no potential, temporary recuperation of the children may be possible, but the long-range benefits arising from education of the mothers will be very limited.

Availability of Other Health or Food Programs. The effectiveness of a Center is almost certain to be enhanced if it is established in a community where it can coordinate its efforts with other health activities or programs for food production. The Center should complement these other services where they exist, and in no case duplicate them.

Cooperation of Local Leaders. Where compatible with the other criteria for selection of communities, the advice of the local leaders will be followed in establishing Centers. Experience with many Centers has shown that lively community interest and involvement is an essential ingredient in the local climate that makes a Center successful. The local leaders can often generate this interest and involvement.

A preliminary survey of a community tentatively selected for a Center is necessary to develop the information on which the decision to locate the Center will hinge. The survey data will also help the organizers and Center personnel in developing the Center to best fit the needs and resources of the community. Equally important, the survey results will help to establish the condition of the community before the Center opens for comparison with its status after the Center has been operating. Following are the major aspects of community life which should be checked.

Identifying the Nutrition Problems. Simple questioning of a 10 percent sample of mothers on the rearing of their children, including weaning practices, foods most prevalent in the diet of children and the amount of food they eat, sanitary practices, and number of children in a family, will provide some of the indications of community nutrition problems. The information gained will help in working out a nutrition education program for mothers that will correct misconceptions and change nutritionally dangerous practices of the community. If it is not possible to make such a study before the Center is put into operation, the questioning can be done as a Center activity during the first week of attendance by the mothers.

Establishing Food Availability and Costs. Accurate surveys of the local market are necessary if a least-cost nutritionally adequate diet for the children is to be developed. Foods having the required nutritional values must be measured accurately so that correct cost/weight figures can be obtained. These surveys have to be done sufficiently in advance of opening the Center so that there will be time to work out appropriate menus.

Establishing the Nutritional Status of Children. Selection of the most malnourished children for first admittance to the Center requires a knowledge of the nutritional status of the preschool children in the community. Where they are available, statistics on births, mortality, and health will give some indications, as will migration patterns and per capita income. Lack of time and personnel may delay gathering this information, but if it can be obtained it will be helpful in understanding the community.

Estimating the Economic Potential. The objectives of the Center will not be attained if the mothers who are educated in nutrition cannot use their education to prevent recurrence of severe malnutrition. Agricultural and economic resources of the community provide valuable indices as to its capacity to fight malnutrition through education. The agricultural resources in a rural area will provide direct means of increasing the availability of protective foods. Semi-industrialization or an adequate labor market in urban areas will provide the purchasing power for the necessary foods. The most valuable sources of information for these data are generally the community leaders and the agricultural extension agents.

If the study of the community potential shows there is a serious doubt as to the ability of three-fourths of the population to put to use the education offered the mothers, other communities should be given priority. If it is decided that a Center is to be established where the potential is below this level, it should from the outset be closely linked with the efforts of other groups to improve the economic conditions of the community.

Determining Extent of Technical Support. Technicians who have already established rapport with the community can provide valuable information and assistance. Social workers and agricultural extension workers, in particular, should be sought out at an early stage in the development of the Center. Their knowledge of the community and acceptance in it can be utilized to good advantage, and coordination with their efforts can be most useful to the Center.

Identifying the Real Leaders. Stimulating the community's interest in a Center can be made easy or difficult by the wielders of influence within the community. It may be a long-term process, however, to identify the leaders and to get them to use their influence on behalf of the Center. Studies made by social scientists, when available, or knowledge gained by other perceptive observers, will help guide the organizers of the Center to the real leaders in the community.

Developing Community Support

The success of a Center depends ultimately on the support of the community, and the support of the community depends on the participation of the community leaders. Even after such participation is secured, it cannot be taken for granted; everything must be done to keep it alive and active.

Informal as well as formal leaders of the community must be identified and motivated so that they can be made active participants. All leaders should be included: the religious leader, the elected official, the sanitary inspector, the teacher, the members of the community action group, and any others who can be identified.

The leaders must be made to understand that their participation is active, energetic, and permanent, and that their collaboration and that of the whole community will consist not only of moral support, but economic assistance and, if necessary, manual labor. It is important, however, that it be made very clear to the leaders that professionally trained people will be in charge of the technical, scientific, and educational aspects of the Center operation.

If there is a Center in operation in a nearby community, the leaders may be made enthusiastic supporters if they are encouraged to visit the Center to see for themselves how such a unit actually operates. Once the interest of the leaders is awakened and their enthusiasm is kindled, they should be encouraged to disseminate their thoughts and feelings throughout the community. Some may not be accustomed to appearing before groups and may need help in presenting their ideas convincingly. It may also be useful at this stage to organize a Pro-Center Council made up of influential members who will represent the community and carry the responsibility for its continuing participation in the activities of the Center.

Community contributions of money, foods, labor, or materials should be carefully registered at the Center so that the use to which they are put and the benefits they provide can be reported to the individual donors or their organizations. In addition, occasions should be created to thank the donors in public, as in church or at community meetings, so that community interest and collaboration can be kept alive.

Recognizing Future Problems

In presenting the Center concept to the leaders and in helping them disseminate their impressions to the community, the organizers must be aware of some of the future problems that may be overcome by recognizing them before the Center is in operation.

Overselling. The benefits of the Center-to-be need to be set forth in realistic terms: better health for the children who attend, the improvement of children's chances to develop their full potential and, for the long range, the benefits the nation can receive from a new kind of citizen. But the Center's limitations must also be set forth clearly. Some children may already be too sick to be saved, some may be so damaged that even if they are saved they may not be able to develop fully; some mothers may not put their knowledge to work and their children may get sick again after leaving the Center. If there is an epidemic, the Center has no miracle cures. These contingencies must be faced and the community must be told that they exist so that if they occur the community will not lose faith in the Center.

The Stigma of Poverty. Extreme care has to be taken to avoid the impression that the selection of children to attend the Center is in any way connected with the poverty of their families. It should be emphasized that the Center does not offer a "feeding" program, but that the children who attend are sick and that their mothers will be taught to use certain foods that should make them well and keep them well—physically and mentally. The educational aspects of the Center's program cannot be overemphasized.

Selecting Housing for the Center

In selecting the housing for the Center the community leaders need to be consulted to avoid stigmas on certain buildings, to provide for construction if necessary, and to encourage their endorsement of the Center's goals. Their recommendations should be followed if they do not conflict with the Center's needs.

Housing for the Center ought to be large enough to accommodate 25 to 30 children and five or six mothers at one time, as well as the Center staff. The physical needs include a food preparation area, an eating area, safe food storage space, an area for children's activities, and sanitary and water facilities appropriate for the community.

Psychological needs of the Center include privacy from other activities and services, visibility to the community, and quarters compatible with the presentation of the Center as a school-type activity rather than a feeding station for malnourished children. A site and building which have some prestige in the community should be chosen, but not at the expense of making the mothers feel insecure in unfamiliar surroundings.

Consideration also has to be given to the length of time the

Center's services are expected to be needed by the population within walking distance. Availability of housing must be assured for that length of time so that it will not be necessary to move the Center once it is established. Where possible, the community's garden area should be close to the Center to encourage contribution of foods. Enough time should be allowed for the selection process so that any construction or remodeling can be completed before the Center opens.

In some areas the Centers have been installed and organized at very low cost by adapting or remodeling nonutilized spaces within or near a health center. This has allowed taking full advantage of common facilities, such as storage space, kitchens, and meeting rooms.

4

Admission and Follow-Up

The system to be used for selection of mothers and children to attend the Center must be decided upon in the early planning of the program. This is a critical part of the program, for if the selection process is explained to the community leaders in advance, later misunderstanding may be prevented. It is important also in the detailed planning which will assure a smooth beginning for the Center.

Certain basic information is needed for the selection process, but its availability and ease of acquisition will vary widely with local conditions.

All children under five years of age in the community should be registered by family. It is helpful to assign a number to the family and to add a suffix number to identify each individual child by his birth order.

In many areas maps of the community are available from community or regional offices or from the malaria eradication agency. Frequently houses will have been numbered for mosquito spraying or address purposes. Such maps and house numbers aid greatly in assuring that a thorough registration of preschool children is carried out.

As each family is registered it is given a family or individual identification card bearing the family number.

It is essential that the central register contain sufficient information to identify and locate all families in the community. The register should provide enough space for the addition of further information from time to time. Where families have clinic or hospital records, the register will show enough information to establish the linkage. Appendix V shows an example of a registration form that has been used successfully in a number of communities in the Philippines.

Birth Dates. It is important to obtain accurate dates of birth of the children registered. Where birth certificates or other records do not exist, an "events calendar" can be prepared, listing the dates of well-known events, such as a hurricane, an election, religious feasts, or the death of an important person. Careful interviews with parents may be able to relate the birth dates of their children with these events.

When it proves impossible to establish even the approximate birth dates, height-weight indices as described in Appendix VIII should be used to identify the most malnourished children.

Weight and Height. Weight and height are critical observations that must be made and recorded carefully during the registration of children. Simple scales that can be carried from house to house can usually be purchased locally. Inexpensive spring scales that can be hung from a tree branch or door lintel are suitable for this purpose, but only if a standard weight is used to check their accuracy on a regular schedule. Height or length of children can easily be determined by use of a simple measuring board.

Signs of Malnutrition. Clinical symptoms of malnutrition are obviously of major importance in the selection of children to be brought to the Center. Edema, or swelling, must be looked for and its distribution noted.* Simple signs of psychomotor development, such as eye-tracking, manual dexterity, and interest in the surroundings, should also be observed and noted.

A number of forms have been developed for the recording of weight and height data, malnutrition symptoms, and signs of psychomotor development, such as the ability to walk, sit, talk, and play. (Samples of forms used in following weight performance are shown in Appendix IV.) These records are essential not only for determining the status of the preschool population for the selection process, but also to provide base line data for evaluation of the children's progress when they attend the Center and after they leave it. The records should provide for observations made at successive intervals over a long period of time.

Criteria for Selection

Medical clearance should be required, when possible, for children with positive skin reactions to tuberculin and for unimmu-

---

* Other classical signs of malnutrition can be learned from study of such texts as D. B. Jelliffe, *The Assessment of the Nutritional Status of the Community,* World Health Organization Monograph Series #53, Geneva, Switzerland, 1966; and Davidson and Passmore, *Human Nutrition and Dietetics,* 3rd edition, Williams & Wilkins, Baltimore, Maryland, U.S.A., 1966.

nized children. A child with primary tuberculosis is almost never contagious but his mother or grandmother may very likely have active, contagious tuberculosis and therefore would be a menace in the Center. If children who have not been immunized against such epidemic diseases as whooping cough, measles, diphtheria, or smallpox are admitted to the Center, the danger of an epidemic must be recognized and a plan of action prepared for this contingency.

Children selected for admission should be in second- and third-degree malnutrition without complications. Those with complications will, of course, be referred for appropriate medical care before the attempt is made to recuperate them and educate their mothers at the Center.

Priority will naturally be given to younger children because after weaning they are more vulnerable to malnutrition and infectious diseases than the older children; they will be selected for earliest admission to the Center. Children less than one year old present special problems and necessitate additional equipment and treatment. If very young children are admitted, the Center will probably need more "baby-sitting" personnel who are alert, kind, and responsible.

The selection of mothers to attend the Center is as important as the selection of children. Those chosen must be willing to accept without reservation the responsibility of getting their children to the Center when they are due, of attending the sessions for which they are themselves scheduled, and of carrying out their assignments while they are at the Center.

Mothers who appear to be ill should be referred for medical clearance rather than risk the infection of the children and other mothers.

In the beginning it is well to consider admitting a few mothers who may be effective in influencing community opinion, even though their children may not be as severely malnourished as some others. The presence in the Center of a wife of a village leader or someone else who is held in high esteem by the community will help in preventing stigmatization of the families who attend the Center.

System of Follow-Up

Follow-up is so crucial to successful recuperation of the children and to reinforcement of the education given the mothers that it must be planned early and explained to the community at the beginning of the program.

Changes in weight and height of the children are the most objective indicators of their nutritional state. Making and recording these observations require no expensive equipment and little sophistication on the part of the observer, and the record system established at the beginning of the program preserves successive measurements for easy reference. The intervals at which the children are weighed and measured during follow-up may be progressively lengthened, provided that their progress is adequate.

Some children will fail to improve in spite of adequate diet; they are almost certain to have other diseases besides malnutrition and should be referred to competent medical facilities for diagnosis and treatment. If a child progresses adequately during his stay in the Center but fails to progress during the follow-up period, a home visit is indicated to determine whether the mother is following the practices learned at the Center.

The attendance of the mothers at the Center may be used as an opportunity to organize them into clubs or alumna groups. Regular meetings can then be planned for the follow-up period. At these meetings the teaching given the mothers is reviewed, with the mothers themselves being induced to do some of the teaching, if possible. Care must be taken to make these meetings vital and enjoyable so that the mothers look forward to them. The activities of the clubs may continue and possibly even be expanded after the Center has been discontinued.

Attention should also be given to the nutritional progress of the younger brothers and sisters of children admitted to the Center. The success or failure of the mothers to nourish their younger children adequately is a rigorous test of the competence they have achieved through their education at the Center.

The mothers may be stimulated to bring their children to the follow-up sessions if a program of immunization or some other service is carried out at these sessions. The physician's explicit interest in their children's state of health is perhaps the strongest positive influence for the mothers' continued cooperation.

5

Evaluating the Results

New ideas in educational techniques and objectives need to be studied when they are first attempted to assess from an unbiased position whether they are well conceived or not. Centers of the kind described here are no exception, and evaluation of their effectiveness has been conducted in a number of countries and is under way in many more. The data available to date on established programs are highly encouraging, verifying that the basic approach is indeed practical as a means of attacking malnutrition in the preschool child.

While testing the validity of the overall approach of the Centers, however, two additional needs for evaluation have become apparent. First, the appropriate kinds of evaluation permit a group starting Centers for the first time to make certain that their operations are going well and to make adjustments before serious troubles develop. Second, even well-established programs involving large numbers of Centers need evaluation as a means of maintaining high performance among the personnel and sustaining support from the communities served by the Centers.

Effectiveness of Maternal Education. The kind of evaluation needed depends upon the aspect of the Center's program that is being considered. The primary objective of the Center is education of the mother through her active participation in the nutritional recuperation of her child. A top priority is the determination of the actual application in the home of what is being taught in the Center. If the evaluation indicates that mothers are not adjusting their child-care practices at home as a result of their experience in the Center, it is obvious that something is seriously amiss.

Adequacy and Acceptability of Menus. Parallel with this objective is the appraisal of the adequacy and acceptability of the menu cycles used in the Centers, because rapid improvement in the child while in the Center is one of the key motivating influences acting on the mothers. Since the menu cycles have been specially developed to allow least-cost but fully adequate nutrition for the child, they are usually rather novel in the dietetic sense, and it becomes extremely important to be absolutely certain of their nutritional adequacy as evaluated by the performance of the children.

In the Center adequate feeding of a child for 50 cents per day is no great feat. At 20 cents per day a little care is involved.

At 15 cents per day the nutritionist-dietitian begins to be challenged. Spending only 12 cents per day is even more of a test, and fully adequate nourishment of a three-year-old on 10 cents per day is something of a dietary victory in most of the world. Centers try to keep the food cost to the absolute minimum consistent with good nutrition so that greater numbers of mothers can be taught to raise healthy children. But it cannot be overemphasized that these least-cost menu cycles need to be carefully evaluated in terms of child response.

Identification of Other Nutritional Deficiencies.   Another objective of evaluation is the identification of new or overlooked nutritional deficiencies in the community. In the preliminary planning for a new Center, base line data are gathered to assess the nature and severity of malnutrition in the community to be served, and the educational emphasis is then fixed to bear on the problems that are encountered. But the situation can change. Drought or hurricane, for example, can alter the food resources of a community abruptly and severely, necessitating adjustment in the thrust of the Center's education. Major changes in land use as a result of agricultural programs can have a similar impact. Then too, in areas where nutritionally important foods are highly seasonal in availability, the timing of the base line studies may have failed to reveal deficiencies that become significant at other times of the year. Evaluation specifically designed to detect these situations is therefore important.

Effectiveness of Personnel.   Because people are human, it should be anticipated that a program of any size covering several years must plan for the continual in-service training of its personnel. Evaluation aimed at estimating the effectiveness of their service and at providing guidance to the supervisors is consequently needed. An example of a report form used for evaluation purposes by nutritionist-dietitians in routine Center visits appears in Appendix IX.

Need to Continue the Center. A program dealing with a number of Centers must anticipate that one of two situations may eventually arise. In small, isolated, immobile communities an effective Center may reach the point where the further educational, public health, and therapeutic benefits of continuing are too small to justify the continued investment of personnel and funds. Evaluation able to detect this point is obviously needed. In unhappier situations, a given Center, for reasons outside the control of the program personnel, may be completely ineffective. Again an evaluation capable of identifying such a situation is required.

Assessing Center Effectiveness

In assessing how well a Center is functioning there are two major categories to be evaluated. One is the response of the children during their participation in the program. The other is the learning of the mothers during their attendance. In measuring these the general experience has been that extensive evaluation of both maternal and child responses is extremely critical in the early phases of Center operations, for it is inevitable that small but important shortcomings will occur and require immediate correction. Later, as the personnel and the community gain experience, a less intensive evaluation is practical.

Child Response. Minimum evaluations of child response while in the Center include accurate measurement of growth. The ideal parameter appears to several experienced groups to be periodic accurate measurement of weight and height and utilization of the height-weight index. Since reference values for what would be expected in terms of the height-weight index are not generally available, these values are included in Appendix VIII along with detailed instructions for their use. A distinct advantage of this system lies in the fact that accurate knowledge of the child's age is not needed, and in many parts of the world accurate data on the age of children cannot be obtained.

An older estimate of growth is determination of the weight of the child, and comparison of this figure with the weight that would be expected for a "normal" child his age. The calculation of this "percent standard weight" is shown in Appendix VIII. In using the percent standard weight it is vital to realize that the child's age must be known to the nearest month.

Further minimum evaluation data include the time required for the clearance of edema, usually a matter of about two weeks in a well-run Center. In addition, careful records should be kept of the frequency and causes of death of any youngsters in the Center. The recording of psychological changes is of value, particularly since these often become apparent before other changes are evident. Stool analyses are also recommended.

The preceding assessments of child response are minimal, particularly in the early stages of Center operations by groups with no previous experience.

In very special situations arrangements may need to be made to do a limited amount of blood and urine analyses to assure that specific problems are being well handled in the Center. For example, in areas with a great deal of beriberi, urinary thiamine analyses will establish quickly whether the menu planning is meeting the problem adequately. In other areas serum vitamin A analyses or determination of serum albumin or hemoglobin may be justified. Once it has become clear that the diets are adequate, however, this kind of evaluation can and should be stopped, simply because Centers are not, in general, research facilities but practical assaults on malnutrition through maternal education and nutritional recuperation of children.

Mother Response. The assessment of the effectiveness of a Center as an instrument of maternal education is unfortunately a more diffuse problem. Nonetheless, determining maternal changes is a matter of first, not second, importance. The most obvious approach, questioning or testing the mothers, has limitations and should never be used as a sole means of evaluation. Yet, testing does reveal one thing: it tells whether the women have learned or failed to learn the child-care facts being taught in the Center. Important points that the mothers are not grasping may indicate the need for new approaches and techniques or merely more repetition.

It must be constantly kept in mind, however, that the goal of the Center is not merely to teach women the facts of improved child care; it is to motivate them to put this new knowledge to regular use in their own homes. There are means of getting at whether this motivation is developing. For example, how frequently do the mothers spontaneously ask questions, and do the questions reveal an increasing understanding of child care and a sense of urgency to do a better job? Is their attitude in the Center one of enthusiastic participation in all of the Center's activities, or is their attendance lackadaisical and casual?

Up-to-date records of attendance by mothers should be kept just as strictly as the attendance records of the children. A low attendance by mothers indicates the need for special efforts towards generating lively interest on their part. Records should be kept, too, of the number of casual visitors coming to the Center with the mothers, because bringing a cousin, a sister, or an older daughter suggests that the mother thinks the Center is an interesting place.

All of these observations on maternal attitude and learning are useful, but they do not constitute the most valid tests of a Center's effectiveness in maternal education. Probably the most meaningful data bearing on this point consist of the results of follow-up studies of the homes to which mother-child pairs return after discharge. If the child himself does not continue to improve or at least hold his own after discharge, something is very wrong, and the cause needs to be sought out. Is the mother just too poor to use what she learned? Has she forgotten something important? Was she simply not motivated? Does the child have some previously unnoticed or new illness? This information is vital, for it can be an invaluable guide to adjustment of Center operations.

While in the home of the discharged mother-child pair it is also useful to assess the nutritional status of the child's brothers and sisters since it is to be hoped that the mother will apply her new knowledge to their care too. It is also valuable, where feasible, to attempt to determine whether there have been improvements in the dietary habits of the family as a whole as a result of the mother's education.

Assessing Impact on Community

Although Centers focus on a relatively small number of mother-child pairs at a time, the cumulative effect of educating succeeding groups should eventually result in significant improvements in the nutritional and overall health status of the community as a whole. In small communities the improvement may be noticeable quite soon, but obviously the greater and the more mobile the population served by a single Center, the longer it will take to see appreciable change. Nonetheless, a program of this kind should ultimately have an influence on overall community nutritional status, and evaluation of the magnitude of these changes is an asset to developing a program of increasing public health significance.

Basic Studies.   For this purpose a number of different kinds of periodic cross-sectional studies are useful. Measurement of the height and weight of the preschool population should eventually show an improvement whether one uses the Gomez classification (Appendix VII), the weight-height index (Appendix VIII), or the weight-for-age distribution (Appendix IV).

There are also a number of vital statistics that are very useful indices of the nutritional status of a population. Wherever possible they should be obtained and, if they are not available, their collection should be urged on local health personnel. These measures include the mortality rate for the ages one to four years; the Wills-Waterlow Index (the mortality rate of children one to four years divided by the mortality rate of infants one to twelve months); morbidity and mortality rates for malnutrition in nearby hospitals; and tabulated causes of death.

There is also a variety of dietary surveys that can be very valuable if the personnel and financial resources are available to obtain the data. Simplest of these is the qualitative food habit survey providing information on what foods are available in the community and in what amounts, since it would be hoped that from the Center would stem an increasing demand for certain particularly nutritious foods. A widespread problem is preferential feeding of adults, particularly men, in the home at the expense of young children. Home visits can be useful to determine if a more reasonable distribution of food within the family is developing as a result of the Center.

More Complex Surveys.   More quantitative and therefore more complex and expensive surveys can generate even more useful data. Maintaining current information on actual food expenditures is extremely helpful because of its direct bearing on menu planning and education at the Center. There are two broad types of dietary survey that can be used, those depending on learning by questionnaire what people have eaten in the previous 24 or 48 hours, and those in which all of the food eaten in the home for a period of several days is weighed. Both types of dietary survey require well-trained, experienced teams if meaningful data are to result, and they are not recommended unless well-trained people are available. Such surveys run by ill-trained personnel can yield grossly misleading results.

It is also important to keep constantly abreast of the enthusiasm of community support for the Center and to devote considerable energy to rekindling of it if it lags.

As general background it is valuable for the Center personnel to keep records of food production changes in the area and to secure estimates of changes in the local sales volume of the food commodities that are being used and recommended in the Center.

Continuing or Terminating a Center

In spite of every effort on the part of the Center staff, the supervisors, and the top echelon people of the program, it is to be expected that occasionally an uncorrectable loss of community interest, or indifference, or even antagonism from community authorities will occur. If every effort to rejuvenate community interest fails, serious thought has to be given to the possible wisdom of moving the Center to an area where more effective work can be done.

Quite a different development needs also to be evaluated when the performance of a Center has been so effective that it has fulfilled its role in education and recuperation and needs to be replaced by other activities in the community. This is a sign of a very good Center that has fulfilled its mission. When this happens thought should be given to moving the Center so that its service can be provided to a community still in need of the kind of assistance these Centers are uniquely suited to provide.

The pertinent data which will indicate that a Center has fulfilled its mission appear to be repeated reselection of the same mother-child pairs, indicating that either those mothers cannot learn or cannot use what they learn; the disappearance of second- and third-degree malnutrition from the preschool-age population; the successful training of essentially all of the mothers in small communities; or failure to observe further improvement in nutritional status in the area of the Center's influence. When these signals appear they indicate that the cost/benefit ratio is becoming excessive as the Center approaches its limits of achievement. Though it will be difficult to abandon a hitherto successful operation, the decision must be made so that the personnel and other resources can be more effectively applied where they are needed more.

The final test of the success of a Center will be the determination that it has done its job so well that it can be closed without harm to its community.

6

A Closing Word

The accumulated experience drawn together now from a dozen countries demonstrates that under a wide variety of circumstances Centers of the type described here can make substantial progress toward eradication of clinical malnutrition among preschool children.

That the Centers accomplish this through maternal education echoes the past decade's urgings of the world's most thoughtful observers of malnutrition: it is only through the mothers that the nutrition of young children can be improved.

While this book concentrates on one general type of practical attack on preschool malnutrition, it is the hope of all the authors that it will also foster other activities capable of making solid progress toward the same goal.

Each of the authors, the participants at the Bogota conference who are listed at the front of this book, has expressed willingness to discuss adaptation of these Centers to any specific local situation about which readers may wish to inquire. Since considerable time has elapsed since the conference, some of the participants may no longer be at the addresses shown. If difficulty is experienced in communicating with any of them, please address inquiries to:

Dr. Sam C. Smith
Chairman, Williams-Waterman Program
Research Corporation
405 Lexington Avenue
New York, New York 10017, U.S.A.

Appendixes

Organizational Charts of Haitian, Colombian, and Philippine Programs

A. Haiti

This program is a government service marked by close collaboration between the Departments of Public Health and Agriculture in rural communities. The effectiveness of this dual direction derives from almost daily discussions between the directors and supporting staff of the two departments. At the community level the agriculturists generate community support for the Center and from the Center gain information on particular families in need of their assistance, and on specific agricultural work that will make the most concrete contribution to the ability of the community to meet its food needs increasingly well. Centers in urban situations are supported exclusively by the Public Health team. Not shown are numerous Centers operated by private, church, and civic groups whose personnel are trained by the Public Health team, and who depend on that team for menu planning and periodic advisory visits.

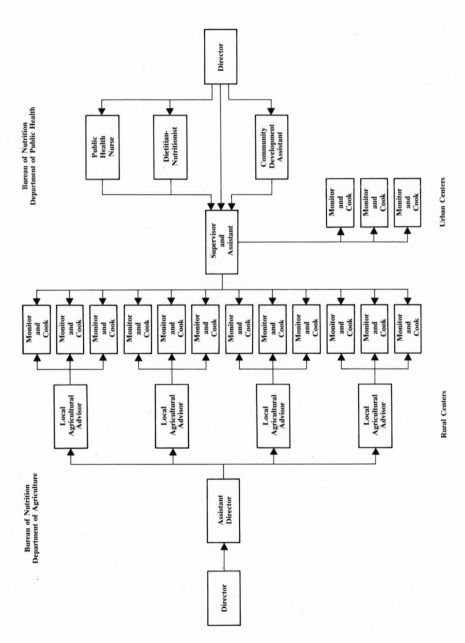

Centers in Colombia are organized and operated jointly by the Sectional Health Services (State Health Services which are connected with the Ministry of Public Health) and the National Institute of Nutrition. In this arrangement each Center is a direct part of a local health program. The Center is considered as an intermediate health service between a hospital pediatric ward and the outpatient clinic of a health center; each center has from three to six satellite Food Demonstration Units in connected health centers of the area. The National Institute of Nutrition promotes and gives economic and technical assistance for the organization and operation of those Centers. This includes seminars and training courses for the health team responsible for the direction of the program or the Center's operation (public health physicians and nurses, pediatricians, auxiliary nurses, baby-sitters, and cooks). The Institute gives permanent supervision through the State PINA Coordinator (public health physician trained in nutrition) and the nutritionist-dietitians of the Applied Nutrition Program. It also supplies the equipment for the Center and the educational material for nutritional education of mothers.

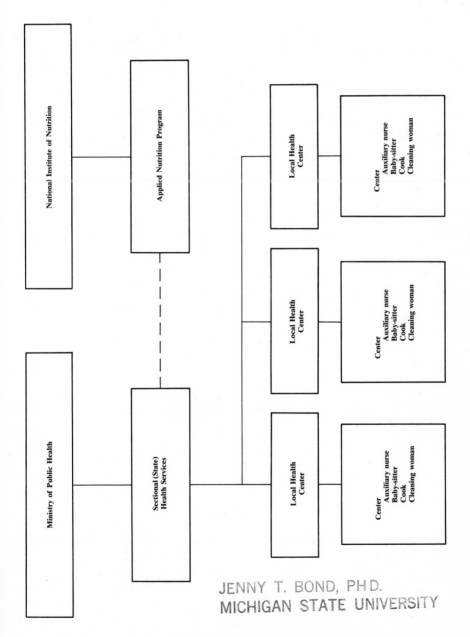

National Institute of Nutrition

Applied Nutrition Program

Ministry of Public Health

Sectional (State) Health Services

Local Health Center

Local Health Center

Local Health Center

Center
Auxiliary nurse
Baby-sitter
Cook
Cleaning woman

Center
Auxiliary nurse
Baby-sitter
Cook
Cleaning woman

Center
Auxiliary nurse
Baby-sitter
Cook
Cleaning woman

The Centers in the Philippines are a formal part of the Public Health program of the Department of Health in collaboration with USAID. In the Philippines a variety of non-governmental and local political groups are relied on in supporting and advisory roles, particularly at the barrio or community level. These include church missions, local nutrition councils, agricultural and social welfare agents, and mayoral offices. Their roles are important, though informal, and not amenable to definition on an organizational chart. The "primary centers" are the fiscal responsibility of the central office while the "secondary centers" are financed totally by local support through the voluntary agencies, and only depend on the national program for training of personnel and technical advice such as equipment selection, menu planning, and daily routine schedules.

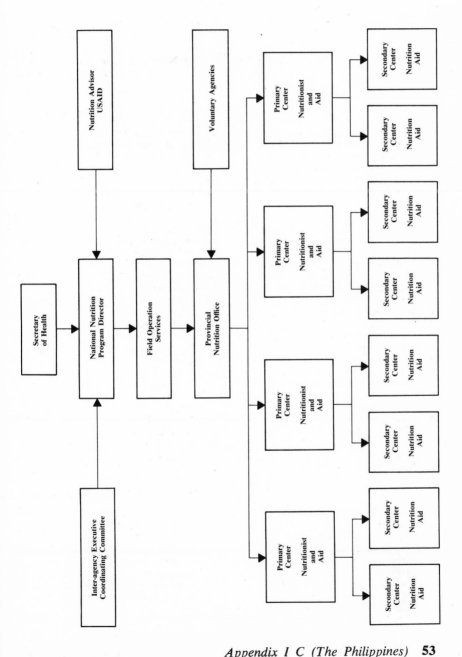

A. **Colombia (20 to 24 Children)**

1	Refrigerator, 12 cubic feet
1	Four-place stove
6	Aluminum pots, size 20–28
1	Aluminum frying pan
2	Aluminum "Olleta" pots for chocolate
1	Wooden cutting board
1	Aluminum grater
1	Sieve, mesh No. 8
1	Large plastic strainer
1	Meat-tenderizing hammer
1	Aluminum pail, 2 gallon capacity
1	Large aluminum basin
1	Large aluminum ladle
1	Large perforated spoon
2	Stainless steel knives
1	Large enamel bowl
1	Medium enamel bowl
1	Food grinder
1	Food scale, 10 kilogram capacity
1	Orange squeezer
1	Wooden beater for preparing chocolate
3	Large wooden spoons
1	Large garbage can
1	Measuring cup
1	Large serving spoon
1	Large serving fork
1	Table for 20 children

20	Chairs for children
2	Metal mesh food covers
1	Aluminum tray
24	Plates
24	Soup bowls
24	Cups
24	Dessert plates
24	Plastic glasses
24	Table servers
2	Aluminum jars
12	Infant bottle feeders
2	Dish racks
1	Blender-mixer
20	Metal cribs
20	Mattresses
48	Pillows
20	Rubber sheets
48	Cotton sheets
48	Cotton pillowcases
20	Blankets
20	Chamber pots
1	Examining table
1	Closet
1	Electric iron
48	Medium bath towels
1	Baby scale
1	Bathroom scale
1	Infantometer (length measurer)

B. **Haiti (30 Children)**

4	Iron cribs with mattresses and covers
4	Large iron pots with lids
2	Pails to carry and store water
3	Large wooden spoons
3	Large metal serving spoons
2	Kitchen knives
2	Aluminum wash basins
30	Plates, deep for dual use as bowls

30	Cups
30	Place settings
1	Table for 30
	Benches to seat 30 children
1	Wooden cutting board
1	Large sieve
1	Scale for weighing children
30	Weight-age forms

Appendix III

Representative Menu Cycles Field-Tested in Brazil, Peru, the Philippines, and Haiti

A. Brazil [19¢ (U.S.) per Child per Day]

Meal	Dishes
Breakfast	Corn meal gruel, coffee
10 a.m. Snack	Seasonal fruit
Lunch	Dry beans and squash Rice Dry salted meat with tomatoes and sweet peppers
2 p.m. Snack	Seasonal fruit
Supper	Vegetable and dry bean soup Cassava (manioc, macaxeira)

B. Peru [20¢ (U.S.) per Child per Day]

Meal	Day 1	Day 2	Day 3
Breakfast	Reconstituted milk Bread Cheese	Reconstituted milk Bread Butter	Reconstituted milk Bread Sweet potato
Lunch	Cucumber salad Carrot soup Stewed fish Rice Watermelon	Fried egg Grits soup Mashed potatoes Rice Pineapple	Fried egg Vegetable soup Stewed beans Rice Papaya
Supper	Hard-boiled egg Vegetable soup Spinach and pota- toes Rice Wheat porridge Reconstituted milk	Mixed salad Oat soup Stew Rice Figs in syrup Reconstituted milk	Vegetable fritters Pumpkin soup Fried beef Rice Figs in syrup Reconstituted milk

C. The Philippines

In these Centers the children are fed half of their daily requirement at the Center, and the mothers are told how to meet the other half at home. These menus range in cost between 2.5¢ and 5¢ (U.S.) per child per day so that the total daily food costs per child per day range from 5¢ to 10¢ (U.S.) if a mother follows Center recommendations.

Day 1   Mongo guisado with ampalaya leaves (mung beans, edible oil, onions, dilis, yellow kamote, ampalaya leaves, and spices)
Chop suey (mung beans, edible oil, onions, tomatoes, beef, carrots, sitsaro, cabbage, and spices)

Day 2   Dried dilis sinigang (mung beans, kamias, rice washings, edible oil, tomatoes, dried dilis, gabi, eggplant, kamote tops, and spices)
Finolang fahong (mung beans, edible oil, onions, tahong, papaya, rice washings, green papaya, malunggay, and spices)

Day 3   Champorado (mung beans, rice, cocoa, sugar, and skim milk powder)
Menudo (mung beans, edible oil, tomatoes, onions, pork, liver, potatoes, and spices)

D.   Haiti [9¢ to 10¢ (U.S.) per Child per Day, Including Fuel]

Meal	*Day 1*	*Day 2*	*Day 3*	*Day 4*
Breakfast	Soup of plantain Sweet potatoes, leaves, ochra, tomatoes, and oil	AK-1000* and pumpkin	AK-1000 and banana	Corn meal and milk
Snack (a.m.)	Fruit juice	Grapefruit juice	Papaya	Mango
Lunch	Pureed pigeon peas, oil, corn meal, and milk	AK-1000, beef-heart, carrots, green beans	AK-1000, liver, cabbage, purselane	Fish-pumpkin puree, AK-1000
Snack (p.m.)	Sweetened milk	Dry skim milk	Dry skim milk	Dry skim milk

*AK-1000 is a local name for a mixture containing 70% corn, millet, or rice and 30% beans. Mothers are taught to make it in their own homes, but a commercial product is also available enriched with niacin, thiamine, riboflavin, iron, and calcium.

Separate growth charts are presented on the following two pages for girls and boys from birth to six years of age; they are adapted from the reference charts used by Dr. Mendez-Castellano in Venezuela.

The top curve on each chart indicates normal expected growth. The next lower curve is 90% of normal. Children falling within this range or above are considered normal. Between the second curve and the third (75% of normal) is first-degree malnutrition. Between the third curve and the fourth (60% of normal) is second-degree malnutrition. Below the bottom curve is third-degree malnutrition.

Individual charts of this kind on which the progress of each child is plotted regularly and discussed with the mother have proven to be useful teaching aids in many countries.

A. Girls' Chart

On the girls' chart is plotted the actual performance of a 29-month-old youngster admitted with second-degree malnutrition, "progressing" to first-degree malnutrition and continuing to respond well in the Center.

B. Boys' Chart

On the boys' chart is plotted the actual record of a 12-month-old child admitted with third-degree malnutrition and edema. The temporary weight loss shown is a result of the disappearance of the edema, following which he moved rapidly into second-degree malnutrition and continued to progress.

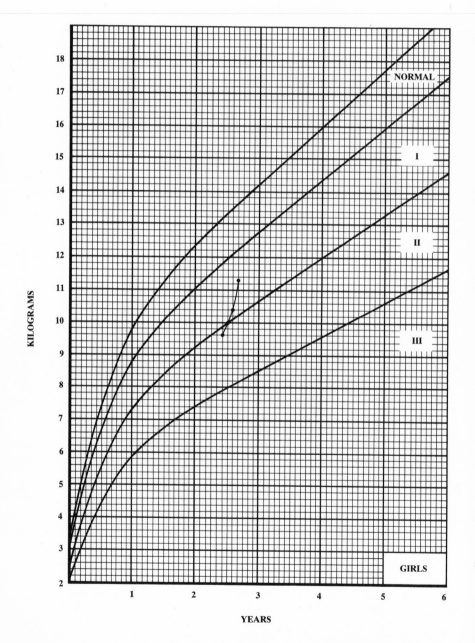

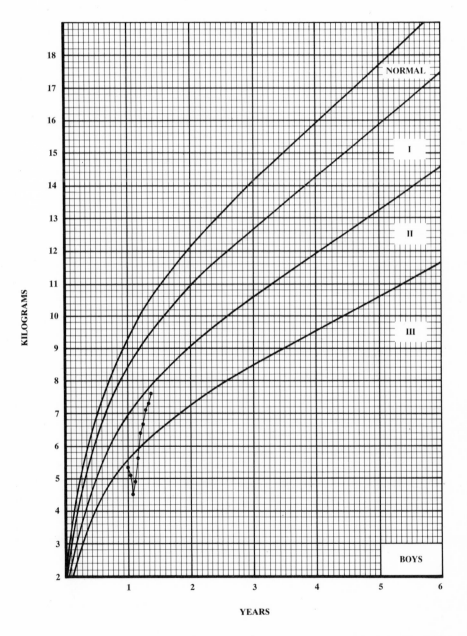

KILOGRAMS

NORMAL

I

II

III

BOYS

YEARS

A simple form used in the Philippines for registering children in a community by family is shown on the opposite page. From the completed forms—which can constitute the central register of all children in the community—it is easy to identify the worst cases of malnutrition and the order in which they may be admitted to the Center.

NATIONAL NUTRITION PROGRAM

Date of Survey _____

Province _____

Municipality _____

Barrio _____

Household No. _____

Father's Name _____

Occupation _____

Mother's Name _____

Occupation _____

CHILD'S NAME	BIRTHDATE	AGE IN MONTHS	WEIGHT (lbs)	STANDARD WT. (lbs)	% NORMAL

Individual Records of Child Performance

A. Weight Record

The least elaborate individual record is that used exclusively to monitor the weight performance of children while they are in the Center and after their discharge. Representative of this kind of record is the Philippine chart shown on the opposite page, duplicates of which allow both the mother and the Central Office to have a record.

B. Health Record

When Centers are affiliated directly with a broader public health program a more detailed record of growth, immunizations, hospitalizations, and out-patient clinic visits is warranted. The individual record form shown on pages 64 through 67 has been found successful with the Centers operated by the Hôpital Albert Schweitzer in Haiti. The top curve on the charts on pages 66 and 67 plots the weight of normal children against age; the bottom curve is about 85% of those normal values. As the individual child's weight is entered on the chart in successive months the resulting curve is easily compared with the reference curves.

NAME _____

DATE OF BIRTH _____

PROVINCE _____

MUNICIPALITY _____

WEIGHT (lbs)

DATE

HEALTH CARD NO. _____

Last Name	First Name

Date of Birth _____ M   F

Mother _____

Father _____

Husband (Wife) _____

Village _____

Neighborhood _____

PHOTO

Typhoid/Paratyphoid A&B	DT	DPT

Smallpox	Polio

Date of First Vaccination:

Reaction:

Measles	BCG	Mantoux

	APPOINTMENTS	
DATE	CLINIC	AUTHORIZATION

HOSPITALIZATIONS OR VISITS TO THE CLINIC

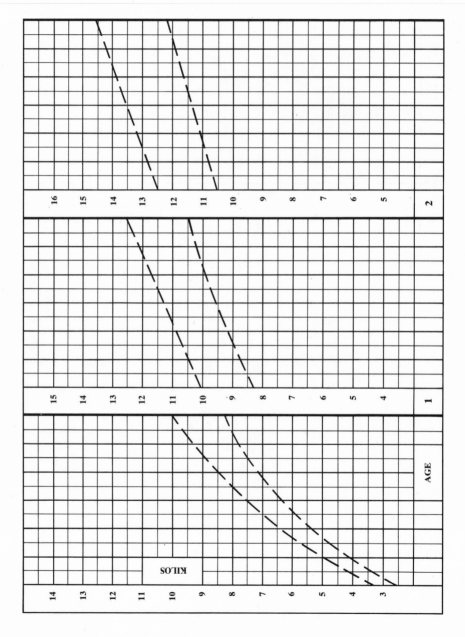

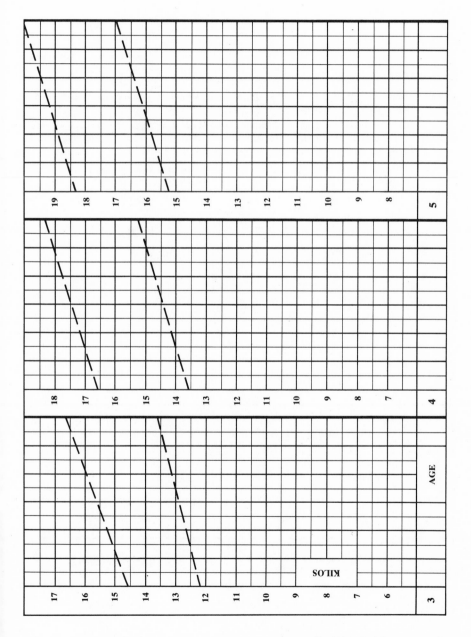

Gomez Classification

This method classifies children according to their weight at a given age compared to that which would be expected.

The "percent standard weight" is calculated as described in Appendix VIII. The child is then classified as "normal," "first-degree malnutrition," "second-degree malnutrition," or "third-degree malnutrition," using the following table.

Range of Percent Standard Weight	Gomez Classification of Degree of Malnutrition
90 or above	Normal
75–89	I
60–74	II
59 or below	III

Percent Standard Weight and Height-Weight Index as Measures of a Child's Growth

These data are derived from measurements of the height and weight of a large group of children from wealthy families in Bogota, Colombia, and can be used as an indication of the pattern of growth to be expected of children receiving good nourishment and good general medical care. These data can be used in two general ways to determine the growth performance of a child.

Percent Standard Weight

When age and weight are known, the "percent standard weight" can be calculated. For example, referring to the table of boys' weights and heights on page 70, a well nourished boy 2 years and 3 months old would be expected to weigh 12.74 kilos. If he weighs only 9.56 kilos his percent standard weight is calculated as follows:

$$\frac{9.56}{12.74} \times 100 = 75\%$$

The objective of a Center, of course, is to *increase* this percentage.

Height-Weight Index

When age cannot be accurately determined, the so-called "height-weight index" can be used. To do this the height in centimeters is divided by the weight in kilograms, and the resulting number or index is compared to that of a well-nourished child of that height. For example, the height-weight index for a boy 91.7 centimeters tall and weighing 10.56 kilos can be calculated as

$$\frac{91.7}{10.56} = 8.68$$

This is in contrast to a normal index as calculated from Appendix VIII A:

$$\frac{91.7}{13.38} = 6.85$$

Here the objective is to *reduce* the index toward the normal.

BOYS—Expected Weight and Height, 0-5 Years

	Age in Years											
	0		1		2		3		4		5	
Months	Weight (kilos)	Height (cm.)	Weight (kilos)	Height (cm.)	Weight (kilos)	Height (cm.)	Weight (kilos)	Height (cm.)	Weight (kilos)	Height (cm.)	Weight (kilos)	Height (cm.)
0	3.260	49.5	9.740	74.7	12.230	86.6	14.130	95.0	15.780	101.9	17.680	107.9
1	4.800	55.2	10.000	75.8	12.400	87.2	14.280	95.6	15.930	102.2	17.860	108.4
2	5.530	58.0	10.240	77.0	12.570	88.2	14.430	96.2	16.080	102.9	18.040	108.9
3	6.170	61.2	10.480	78.1	12.740	88.9	14.570	96.8	16.230	103.2	18.220	109.4
4	6.750	63.2	10.700	79.2	12.900	89.6	14.710	97.4	16.380	104.0	18.400	109.8
5	7.240	64.8	10.900	80.2	13.060	90.3	14.840	98.0	16.540	104.3	18.590	110.3
6	7.700	66.7	11.100	81.2	13.220	91.0	14.970	98.5	16.700	104.9	18.780	110.7
7	8.110	68.0	11.300	82.2	13.380	91.7	15.100	99.1	16.860	105.5	18.970	111.2
8	8.500	69.5	11.500	83.2	13.530	92.3	15.230	99.7	17.020	105.9	19.160	111.6
9	8.850	71.0	11.700	84.1	13.680	93.0	15.360	100.2	17.180	106.2	19.350	112.0
10	9.170	72.2	11.880	85.0	13.830	93.7	15.500	100.8	17.340	106.9	19.540	112.5
11	9.460	73.5	12.060	85.9	13.980	94.3	15.640	101.2	17.510	107.4	19.730	112.9

GIRLS—Expected Weight and Height, 0-5 Years

Age in Years

Months	0 Weight (kilos)	0 Height (cm.)	1 Weight (kilos)	1 Height (cm.)	2 Weight (kilos)	2 Height (cm.)	3 Weight (kilos)	3 Height (cm.)	4 Weight (kilos)	4 Height (cm.)	5 Weight (kilos)	5 Height (cm.)
0	3.000	48.4	9.280	73.5	11.870	84.9	13.700	93.7	15.340	100.8	17.210	107.1
1	4.160	53.8	9.550	74.6	12.030	85.8	13.840	94.3	15.480	101.2	17.390	107.6
2	4.930	56.4	9.810	75.6	12.190	86.5	13.980	95.0	15.620	101.9	17.570	108.1
3	5.600	60.0	10.060	76.6	12.350	87.3	14.120	95.6	15.760	102.4	17.750	108.6
4	6.200	62.0	10.300	77.7	12.510	88.1	14.260	96.2	15.910	103.0	17.930	109.1
5	6.730	64.0	10.530	78.7	12.670	88.8	14.390	96.8	16.060	103.5	18.110	109.6
6	7.200	65.6	10.750	79.6	12.830	89.5	14.520	97.4	16.210	104.0	18.300	110.0
7	7.640	67.1	10.960	80.6	12.980	90.3	14.650	98.0	16.370	104.6	18.490	110.3
8	8.030	68.5	11.160	81.2	13.130	90.9	14.780	98.6	16.530	105.1	18.680	110.9
9	8.370	69.8	11.350	82.2	13.280	91.6	14.920	99.1	16.700	105.6	18.870	111.4
10	8.690	71.1	11.530	83.3	13.420	92.3	15.060	99.7	16.870	106.1	19.070	111.9
11	8.990	72.4	11.700	84.2	13.560	93.0	15.200	100.3	17.040	106.6	19.270	112.3

Appendix IX

Check List for Supervisor Visits

This sample check list is adapted from the one used in Haiti when the supervisor visits Centers to evaluate the overall operation.

Report on Status of Center at _____ date _____

	Good	Passable	Poor	Not Observed
Cleanliness of Tables				
In the kitchen area	☐	☐	☐	☐
In the eating area	☐	☐	☐	☐
Condition of plastic tablecloth	☐	☐	☐	☐
Thorough Use of Disinfectants				
In the kitchen area	☐	☐	☐	☐
In the eating area	☐	☐	☐	☐
Cleanliness of Floors				
In the kitchen area	☐	☐	☐	☐
In the eating area	☐	☐	☐	☐
In the house in general	☐	☐	☐	☐
Use of disinfectant	☐	☐	☐	☐
Use of soap	☐	☐	☐	☐
Use of clean water	☐	☐	☐	☐
Condition of brooms	☐	☐	☐	☐
Condition of pail or bowl	☐	☐	☐	☐
Cleanliness of Center Facility				
Kitchen closets orderly and clean	☐	☐	☐	☐
Hall and house closets orderly and clean	☐	☐	☐	☐
Foyer solid and safe	☐	☐	☐	☐
Foyer clean	☐	☐	☐	☐
Pantry arrangement	☐	☐	☐	☐
Pantry cleanliness	☐	☐	☐	☐
Fuel storage orderly	☐	☐	☐	☐
Fuel utilization economy	☐	☐	☐	☐
Handling of Table and Cooking Ware				
Washing of tableware	☐	☐	☐	☐
Washing of utensils	☐	☐	☐	☐
Washing of pots for boiling water	☐	☐	☐	☐
Use of soap	☐	☐	☐	☐
Use of clean water	☐	☐	☐	☐
Rinsing of tableware and utensils	☐	☐	☐	☐

	Good	Passable	Poor	Not Observed
Handling of Table and Cooking Ware (continued)				
Water storage equipment	☐	☐	☐	☐
Drying of tableware	☐	☐	☐	☐
Disposal of Garbage				
Frequency of disposal	☐	☐	☐	☐
Mode of disposal: burned	☐	☐	☐	☐
buried	☐	☐	☐	☐
other	☐	☐	☐	☐
Number of flies	☐	☐	☐	☐
Use of flypaper	☐	☐	☐	☐
Use of insecticide	☐	☐	☐	☐
Latrines				
Regular washing	☐	☐	☐	☐
Regular use by children old enough	☐	☐	☐	☐
Regular use of hygienic paper	☐	☐	☐	☐
Food Preparation				
Peeling of vegetables	☐	☐	☐	☐
Peeling of fruits	☐	☐	☐	☐
Length of cooking	☐	☐	☐	☐
Quantity of water used	☐	☐	☐	☐
Meals				
Schedule of feeding: breakfast	☐	☐	☐	☐
snack	☐	☐	☐	☐
dinner	☐	☐	☐	☐
snack	☐	☐	☐	☐
Time allowed for eating	☐	☐	☐	☐
Care of Children				
Handwashing after toilet	☐	☐	☐	☐
Handwashing before breakfast	☐	☐	☐	☐
Cleanliness of nails	☐	☐	☐	☐
Bathing of children before dinner	☐	☐	☐	☐
Cleanliness of bathing water	☐	☐	☐	☐
Convenience of soap to bathing	☐	☐	☐	☐
Education of Mothers				
Participation in preparation	☐	☐	☐	☐
Participation in cooking	☐	☐	☐	☐
Participation in serving meals	☐	☐	☐	☐
Frequency of instruction of mothers	☐	☐	☐	☐
Factual knowledge of mothers	☐	☐	☐	☐
Interest, complaints, and requests of mothers (list separately)	☐	☐	☐	☐

	Good	*Passable*	*Poor*	*Not Observed*
Bookkeeping				
Menus	☐	☐	☐	☐
List of purchases	☐	☐	☐	☐
Mothers' attendance for service	☐	☐	☐	☐
Mothers' attendance at general meetings	☐	☐	☐	☐
Attendance of children	☐	☐	☐	☐
Incidence of contagious or other sicknesses	☐	☐	☐	☐
Weight records of children	☐	☐	☐	☐
Weekly reports	☐	☐	☐	☐

Health Problems

Diarrhea: number of cases _____
           serum prepared,   yes ☐   no ☐
           sulfaguanidine given,   yes ☐   no ☐

Fever: number of cases _____
        treated with aspirin,   yes ☐   no ☐

Sores and burns: number of cases _____
           adequate treatment,   immediate ☐   delayed ☐
           superficial treatment,   yes ☐   no ☐

Lack of appetite: number of cases _____
           milk supplement given,   yes ☐   no ☐